# OUTLAST

The science and craft of life span

By

## Michael P. Shea

# Table of contents

# DISCLAIMER

# Introduction

Cancer, heart disease, and type 2 diabetes are just a few of the life-threatening conditions that have emerged in our modern world. In addition, despite the fact that our modern lifestyle is superior to that of our ancestors, some aspects of our environment are putting our health at risk.

Our environment has changed a lot over the past few centuries, but our genes have not. This is the main problem. Take fructose, for instance. It used to be our companion when it came to products of the soil, yet presently it's wherever in our food, making us store more fat than we really want. What's more, it's not simply current food that is not perfect for our well-being - the amount we move, our rest propensities, and, surprisingly, the impact of virtual entertainment on our feelings are having a significant cost. So we really want to concoct a strategy to live well in this bizarre new world.

A comprehensive guide to living a longer, healthier, and more satisfying life is Outlive (2024). Drawing on state-of-the-art science and useful exhortation, it enables you to improve your activity, nourishment, rest, and profound well-being for the most extreme life span.

# Chapter 1

## A competitor of life

You've likely known about the many advantages of ordinary activity. Be that as it may, do you have any idea how significant it is for carrying on with a long life? Indeed, it just so happens, that even a tad of activity can have an enormous effect. Besides the fact that exercise fortifies your heart and muscles - it further develops course and advantages your cerebrum by delivering a particle called BDNF - mind-determined neurotrophic factor - which assists with memory.

With everything taken into account, practice resembles this mystical elixir that can assist you with living longer, better lives, and it's not even about picking sides between cardio or loads - everything no doubt revolves around finding exercise propensities that work for you exclusively.

Presently, here's the astounding part - even only a tad piece of normal activity can have a gigantic effect and really stretch your life by quite a while, postpone ongoing illnesses, and, surprisingly, dial back or opposite mental deterioration. Basically going from zero to an hour and a half seven days can bring down your gamble of biting the dust for any reason by 14%!

What's more, obviously, being really fit implies you're considerably less liable to bite the dust than if you're a habitually lazy person. Concentrates on showing that the fittest individuals have the most minimal death rates. As a matter of fact, having a low degree of cardiorespiratory wellness is more hazardous than smoking.

Here is a great method for pondering remaining dynamic as you age: become a life-long athlete! Envision you're preparing for a centenarian decathlon, a rundown of ten actual errands you need to have the option to do when you're 100 years of age. These may be climbing steps, getting up off the floor, or climbing a path. This will assist you with defining objectives for your wellness process and keep you roused.

Therefore, select your ten events and begin preparing for them. Everything without question revolves around being balanced and remaining dynamic in various ways. Like that, you'll be considerably more prone to be fit and solid at 100 years of age - and break the generalization that advanced age must be about decline and hopelessness.

# Chapter 2

# The three components of wellness

So now that you know the significance of a deep-rooted love of activity, we should get into certain points of interest that you can apply to your preparation routine. There are three critical elements of wellness - high-impact perseverance and proficiency, strength, and soundness. Train around there must keep up with well-being and strength as you age.

Oxygen-consuming perseverance and productivity can be improved by preparing with zone 2 cardio, a particular power level that can be supported for longer periods. This suggests a moderate power level, typically expecting 60 to 70 percent of your greatest pulse. At the end of the day, going on like this, you should in any case pretty much have the option to hold a discussion yet most certainly not sing a power song.

This kind of preparation advances involving fat as fuel and is significant for nonathletes, as it fabricates perseverance and forestalls ongoing illnesses. An illustration of zone 2 preparation is strolling energetically for six to ten miles day to day. Two 30-minute sessions per week can provide significant benefits as a starting point. To make zone 2 preparation more charming, have a go at paying attention to webcasts or book recordings during your exercises.

Next up are $VO_2$ max exercises - these are instructional meetings intended to build the greatest measure of oxygen that your body can use during exercise. This kind of activity ordinarily includes stop-and-go aerobic exercise, also called HIIT. What precisely is that? In HIT, you switch back and forth between times of focused energy exercise and rest.

Additionally, HIT is related to life span and useful limit. To get everything rolling, have a go at enhancing zone 2 work with a couple of $VO_2$ max exercises each week, consisting of spans enduring three to eight minutes at the most extreme reasonable speed, trailed by simple activity.

It's significant not to disregard strength with regards to workout - it's critical for safeguarding against actual delicacy and injury in advanced age. Bulk and bone thickness decline over the long haul, so it's crucial to consolidate weighty obstruction preparing to further develop muscle filaments and keep up with bone wellbeing. Practices like rucking - climbing with a stacked rucksack - or conveying weighty metal loads can assist with fortifying the body.

To wrap things up, grasp strength is a fundamental part of generally speaking strength and is likewise connected to life span. To further develop hold strength, attempt practices like rancher's conveys and dead-swinging from a draw-up bar. Additionally, centers around offbeat strength and pulling movements, as well as hip-pivoting developments like single-leg step-ups and split-position Romanian deadlifts. That could seem like a ton to take in, so most certainly gain these activities from an educated mentor or utilize educational recordings as an asset.

By integrating these preparation strategies and zeroing in on high-impact perseverance, strength, and solidness, you can get yourself positioned for a satisfying and dynamic life as you age.

# Chapter 3

## Patching up your eating routine

Since you have your activity routine cut out for you, we should change gears and investigate everything about our diet. A major issue Americans face these days is known as the Standard American Eating routine, or Miserable. It's stacked with sugar, refined carbs, and handled oils, which can prompt indulging and chronic weakness. To break liberated from the Miserable snare, you can attempt caloric limitation, dietary limitation, or time limitation. Keep in mind that each approach has its advantages and disadvantages, so pick what accommodates your way of life best.

The caloric limitation is the most adaptable choice yet requires following all that you eat and fighting the temptation to swindle. Dietary limitation includes cutting explicit food sources yet possibly works on the off chance that it prompts a calorie deficiency. Time limitations, such as discontinuous fasting, can misfire if you gorge or don't get sufficient protein.

We should flip this around briefly and change the concentration to what you ought to eat. First up is protein - it's fundamental for building and keeping up with muscle, particularly as we age. Go for the gold one gram of protein for every pound of body weight day to day, or 2.2 grams per kilo. Spread your protein admission over the day, and pick excellent sources like whey protein confine over soy protein disengage. Eating sufficient protein can likewise assist you with feeling full, so you'll consume fewer calories generally. Keep in mind that protein helps you feel full and keep up with bulk, particularly as you age. Keep in mind that protein from animals is more effective than protein from plants.

Fats are next. Not all fats are made equivalent! We want a blend of immersed, monounsaturated, and polyunsaturated fats, with an emphasis on omega-3s for heart and mind wellbeing. Reduce your intake of butter, lard, and omega-6-rich oils like corn, soybean, and sunflower, as well as nuts and extra virgin olive oil.

Fasting, or eating under strict time constraints, can be beneficial, but not for everyone. There are momentary eating windows, substitute-day fasting, and longer-term fasting. Irregular fasting and time-confined eating are famous weight reduction strategies, yet their adequacy and potential drawbacks are disputable. Fasting triggers physiological and cell systems like insulin level drops and cell fix quality initiation. However, prolonged fasting may result in muscle loss. Having said all that, fasting can work for weight reduction, however, it should be drawn nearer with wariness and accuracy. Counseling your PCP before starting a fasting regimen is presumably best.

Finally, we should discuss taking on what Attia calls a Nourishment 3.0 mentality. Everything revolves around tracking down the right equilibrium that works for you. Focus on reducing overall energy intake, getting enough protein, and finding the right fat-fat ratio instead of overthinking it. Additionally, recollect that activity and investing energy outside are similarly significant for your well-being. Eventually, there's nobody-size-fits-all methodology, so it depends on you to track down your equilibrium.

# Chapter 4

# The power of sleep

Now that you know how to exercise and eat right, it's time to learn how much sleep affects your health and well-being. After coming close to death, Attia realized how important sleep is for both physical and mental health. After going without sleep for 60 hours, he fell asleep behind the wheel, narrowly avoiding a serious car accident. This nerve-racking experience ought to act as a strong wake-up call for everybody to rethink their relationship with rest and focus on it as a fundamental part of a sound way of life.

Stories to the side, there are a lot of examinations showing the adverse consequences of an absence of rest - to be sure, it's been connected to an expanded gamble of things like coronary failures, type 2 diabetes, and even working environment mishaps. It's not just about feeling tired - it's about your general wellbeing. For instance, one review showed that dozing under seven hours a night can build your gamble of biting the dust rashly by 12%. Sleep deprivation also contributes to an increase in workplace accidents and medical errors, as evidenced by the fact that sleep-deprived drivers are responsible for approximately 20% of all car accidents.

However, let's shift gears and return to the positive aspects. Studies have shown that we want around seven and a half to eight-and-a-half long periods of rest every evening. With great rest, your physical and mental presentation can improve, including things like athletic execution and memory union. In addition, getting enough sleep helps regulate your metabolism and lowers your risk of developing chronic health issues like metabolic dysfunction, type 2 diabetes, heart disease, and obesity.

Many individuals look for that enchanted pill to make it lights-out time for them, yet actually, many tranquilizers out there don't further develop the best quality. Some, like Ambien and Valium, can even disrupt your sleep. So, what can you do to naturally improve your sleep?

In the first place, it's fundamental to assess your rest propensities. Use rest trackers or take rest polls like the Pittsburgh Rest Quality Record to sort out how you're doing. Remember, everybody's unique - a few of us are morning individuals, while others are evening people. Along these lines, attempt to work with your regular beat.

Presently onto a few additional substantial tips. It's certainly smart to eliminate blue light openness before bed, perhaps by trading out those Drove bulbs for hotter ones. Keep your room cool, around 65 degrees Fahrenheit or 18 degrees Celsius - and ensure your room is pretty much as dull as could be expected. Attempt to stay away from screens an hour before sleep time - that late-night virtual entertainment scroll isn't making a difference.

- Be aware of what you consume, as well. Hold caffeine and liquor under wraps, as they can screw with your rest. Lastly, remember to oversee pressure - contemplation can be a unique advantage for slowing down.

Indeed, even hotshot competitors like LeBron James focus on rest for maximized operation. He purportedly dozes around 12 hours every day with an extraordinary sleeping pad and cushions! In this way, remove a page from LeBron's playbook and make a rest schedule that works for you. Stick to it, and you'll be

headed to more readily rest and work on

generally speaking prosperity.

# Chapter 5

## Embracing profound wellbeing

You've arrived at the last part of your life span - close to home wellbeing. You probably focus on your physical health when you think about being healthy, but your emotional health is just as important, if not more so. All things considered, what benefit is carrying on with a long life if you're unsettled or satisfied?

For instance, somebody battling with wretchedness probably won't see the purpose in getting a disease screening or checking their glucose levels. Then again, somebody who's in great shape probably won't understand what intense subject matters can mean for their general well-being. In this way, assuming you're managing close-to-home or psychological well-being battles, go ahead and provide proficient assistance. It's urgent to resolve these issues to keep up with great actual well-being.

Managing close-to-home well-being can be interesting. In contrast to physical health, it is difficult to identify and diagnose. That is the reason you want a proactive and individualized approach. Pay special attention to indications of profound medical problems, look for help early, and focus on everyday practices that advance long haul close to home prosperity.

There are various instruments to screen and keep up with close-to-home harmony. Prescriptions, contemplation, and hallucinogens can help, yet they're not handy solutions. They ought to be viewed as a component of genuine psychotherapy, as rationalistic conduct treatment or DBT. This is a demonstrated technique that controls feelings and endures close-to-home stressors. DBT is based on four points of support: close-to-home guidelines, trouble resilience, relational viability, and self-administration, all connected to care. However, it is essential to keep in mind that transformation takes time and effort. Rehearsing every day and taking care of problems with treatment is vital to accomplishing genuine recuperation.

Something else to consider is self-reflection. Many individuals battle with self-loathing and the requirement for outside approval. It's crucial to work on your relationship with yourself and perceive how your previous encounters shape your current way of behaving. Take adolescent injury, for example. It can appear in different structures, similar to compulsion, codependency, and relational issues. It's critical to resolve such issues, yet this can be a genuine test. So what else is there to do? Be on the lookout for clues that something is wrong with your emotional health, get help right away, and make a point to practice meditation or self-reflection every day. What's more, recall, recuperating takes time, so show restraint toward yourself during the cycle.

In conclusion, how about we return to life span? Focus on the future and pursue your goals and dreams if you want to remain healthy and "young." Find exercises that give you pleasure and satisfaction, such as investing energy in nature, rehearsing care, or journaling.

Keep in mind, that close-to-home well-being is similarly pretty much as significant as actual well-being. Take care of yourself, and if you need it, don't be afraid to ask for help. With time, persistence, and the right devices, you can gain ground toward a more joyful and better life.

# Conclusion

Working out, a fair eating routine, quality rest, and profound well-being are vital parts of living a more extended, better life. The practice works on your dissemination and cerebrum capability, while a balanced eating regimen, including protein, solid fats, and caloric limitation, can assist you with keeping up with bulk and by and large well-being. Focusing on your rest and making a steady standard advances physical and mental execution. Your profound well-being is comparably crucial, and resolving issues like discouragement or injury can add to your general prosperity. By zeroing in on this large number of regions, you can make progress toward a satisfying, dynamic, and sound life.

www.ingramcontent.com/pod-product-compliance
Lightning Source LLC
Chambersburg PA
CBHW070756260726
48660CB00007B/3151